Are Prescription Drugs Really Safe?

A summarized expert review on drug safety
written for everyone to understand

by Dr. Vera M. Madzarevic

Third Edition

Table of Contents

Acknowledgements

I want to especially thank to my family who are always open for discussion, supportive and very critical of my work.

I also want to acknowledge my English proof-reader Miss Dina Miovic, who took the time and effort to not only correct the English style, but to provide valuable critical insight on how to simplify concepts to make them really uncomplicated for everyone to understand.

Also, I want to thank everyone I met in my lifetime since they left an impression, which impression made me who I am, and further who I ought to become.

Preface to the third edition

Empowering patients on treatment options allows the proper understanding of expectations and enables active participation in health care decisions. One component of empowerment is information. Understanding what drugs safety is, promotes better treatment conformity and facilitates the recognition of side effects that may become a serious issue. This book contains information every person that is taking either prescription or over the counter medications should have access to. Drug safety is ultimately the most important goal of the pharmaceutical industry, but what does it means for ordinary people? One of the issues regarding drug safety is that drug information on their safety and efficacy in lay language is scarce and not easy accessible. It is not always easy to understand what drug safety means and how it can affect your life. This book provides patients with a simplified approach to drug safety. Concepts are clearly presented, easy to read and with take away points were incorporated to allow further reference. The topics covered include: • The drug safety concept • Brief history of drug development • The randomized controlled clinical trial and evidence based medicine • Risk/benefit assessment and how the decision is made • Drug effects, benefits • Variability in drug response • Personalized medicine and patient centered care • Drug tolerance • Side effects • Participation in treatment decisions • Quality of life • Compliance to treatment • Drugs with special pharmacology • Pharmacogenomics • Dose, dosage, and length of treatment • Dosage forms • Off label use • Slow release/timed release/extended release forms.

As a continuous improvement process, I update the book once more to give you the most current information on drug safety and health care. I even shortened the title to make it easier to buy.

In this revision, I included three concepts of health care and medicine that creates confusion when discussed and presented as a new solution to you. Therefore, I included a detailed review of Patient Centered Medicine vs. Patient Centric Medicine and vs. Personalized Medicine.

Dr. Vera Madzarevic
February 10, 2016, Toronto, Canada

Preface to the second edition

Once completed the first edition, I wanted to further test the readability and clarity of the book.

The result was amazing. The opinion of the readers was very encouraging. They suggested highlighting the main concepts and creating take away points to provide an easy access resource where the reader can refer to very easily. Although this is not a text book, it intends to be informative and educative.

I also added two more chapters where off-label use of marketed drugs and safety concerns regarding slow/ timed/ extended release forms are discussed.

Vera M. Madzarevic
October 3, 2014
Toronto, Canada

Preface

I wrote this book because I wanted to bring some light to the concept of drug safety to the general public. When I first started thinking about the concept of the book, my first challenge, and my top priority, was to write it in such a manner so as to both make it easy and simple to read, as well as to provide the reader with key information there is to know before making the decision to take a specific drug. It was of utmost importance to me to achieve that you have understood all the main concepts well, so you could have a better insight into the medication you are taking.

This book does not intend to replace your doctor's opinion or make any diagnosis or recommend treatment of your disease. You must always contact your health care provider before introducing any changes into your medication.

Also, this book does not intend to point fingers or "uncover" the hidden truths about drugs, because there are none. Generally, most of the information about all prescription medication out there on the market is readily available. All that information was/has been gathered over the years of clinical development, with the investment of almost two billion US dollars yearly per new drug and with the participation of thousands of patients. The reality is that the information we, clinical scientists, acquire, and the information that pharmaceutical companies provide, are seldom read, unless you are the regulator or the competitor.

I personally am amazed every time we test a drug and observe how the human body reacts to, uses and gets rid of it. It is remarkable how our bodies are able to absorb, distribute, metabolize and readily eliminate drugs as well as any foreign substance!

We are basically the result of our genetic makeup, our interaction with our environment and the way we were nurtured. The interaction with our environment includes what we eat and drink, where we live and how our body adapts to it. Due to all these reasons, those tiny differences that make us unique are enough to affect our response to drugs.

Let me tell you the story of how I choose to dedicate my life to discovering and developing new therapies.

When I was very little I recall being very sick. My tonsils were often infected, and my nose was filled with polyps. With the best of their intentions, doctors kept prescribing me antibiotics, antihistamines, and pain relievers. I recall all those medications, packed by the manufacturer in boxes that contained a leaflet with lots of information written in a very small font and on very thin paper. I could barely read, I could not understand a word, it was complicated. I used to keep the leaflets in a spiral binder for my own personal collection, so one day I would be able to read and understand the information they contained. I also kept asking myself how they discovered the way the stomach reacts to a drug. How did they ask the stomach? The stomach cannot speak...

Another big question I had in my head was how come my brother, who was twice my size and weight, was prescribed the same antibiotics in the same dose as myself. Shouldn't I get less, or he more?

For years I wondered if the medications I was taking were really safe. I knew a lot about side effects, and I had almost all of them, including diarrhea, headache, dizziness, redness and flushing, metallic taste, nausea, heartburn, allergies, and even once my kidneys hurt. When I was a little kid, nobody asked me how I felt after taking a medication, nor if I was happy with my quality of life. The reality was that in the 1960s, children were seldom part of clinical trials. There were no controlled data available to support the safety and efficacy of medications in children. All that has changed now, and presently drugs that include children in their labelling must have clinical trial data in the children population to support their safety and efficacy.

It is also astonishing how much medications have improved our lives. I have my little story on that one, too. I remember vividly the day Apollo 11 reached the moon and the first moonwalk, as it was transmitted on TV. I even remember the last names of the astronauts: Armstrong, Aldrin and Collins. I was very sick around that time, lying in bed with my tonsil infection again. On that day, my parents took me out of bed to the dining room where the TV set was. They lied me down onto the dining table, and gave me a children's aspirin (the little pink pill that tasted like strawberries). Dad told me...``Vera, we are sorry for waking you up and taking you out of bed, but today humanity is making history, and we want you to be part of it. Thanks to the aspirin I took, I was feeling better enough for long enough a time so as to be able to witness that historical moment. The point of the story is that, if I hadn't taken that medication, I would have missed out on something important in

16

my life that I would have later surely regretted, as the man's walk on the moon was unfortunately never repeated in almost 50 years that had passed since.

In that moment, I made the decision that I, too, wanted to make a difference in human lives and help fight suffering. I wanted to be a doctor and find new medical miracles in order to help people live better lives. Of course, nobody in my family believed me at that point, they thought I was too small to even think like that. Nevertheless, I had an objective and I worked towards it regardless of all the obstacles I was yet to overcome.

I must assert that thanks to the pharmaceutical industry and drug research in general, despite all the negative thoughts we may have about them, they must be credited for improving the lives of billions of people worldwide. We have the largest world population ever recorded, and growing. We live longer and healthier lives. Of course, as is the case with any business, there are some really great pharmaceutical companies, and then there are those others that are not worth mentioning.

Unfortunately, one bad example is often enough to tarnish the entire industry.

Our health is the most precious thing we have, and we should be able to access all information, without restrictions, about the safety and efficacy/efficiency of the drugs we take through better transparency rules. It is time that patient empowerment joined forces with education, information, knowledge and choice. Regulators and stakeholders have taken this very seriously and there is more transparency in this field now than there has ever been before. This will allow independent reviews of raw data, by different groups of scientists, to further verify safety and efficacy of marketed drugs.

By now, you probably have a clear idea of what the aim of this book is, and were also able to calculate my age. After this overview, we will enter together the amazing world of concepts in pharmacology made easy. Come on in, turn the page.

Vera M. Madzarevic
July 4, 2014 Venice, Italy.

Introduction

Just recently, I was reviewing the FDA[1] Med-Watch reports on safety issues concerning market-ed drugs in the United States, and started thinking that despite the best efforts of the regulators in the US, Canada and Europe, patients are seldom informed promptly, if ever, about serious safety concerns regarding the very same drugs that they are being prescribed.

It is my opinion that patients should actively participate in the decision regarding taking a medication if serious safety concerns exist.

The pharmaceutical industry invests billions of dollars on research and development every year, provide all the information as obtained in clinical trials in order for the regulators to review, and now even make them available for other scientists to make independent reviews, and still, emergency rooms are filled with patients who developed serious side effects or even died because of pre-scribed medications used, in general, within the safety parameters established by the manufacturer. We are all very familiar with the cases of several

---

[1] FDA - US Food and Drug Administration

celebrities who lost their lives due to prescription drugs use or misuse. So where is the problem?

It is not an easy answer, since there are many factors that play a crucial role in this catastrophe of widespread proportions.

Throughout the 17 chapters in this book, I will walk you through many concerns and issues that you have to know about before you take a drug. Ultimately, your health is in your hands.

Please do note that I deliberately use the word 'drug' as an abbreviated version of the word/ phrase 'prescription drug', or 'medication', to simplify the reading.

1

Underlining some important issues

One of the issues I can very easily point out to is that, despite the fact that there is an ocean of data available on the Internet, there isn't enough information on the safety and efficacy of medications available in lay language, and if there is, it is not easily accessible. Another issue regarding drug information is that it has to be qualified before you can make any rational use of it in the process of making your decision about taking a drug. (as a decision-making tool)

The term 'qualifying drug information' implies establishing the source of the said information about a specific drug as valid and truthful. An example of a valid and truthful source of information about drugs is for example the FDA or other regulatory agency web site. Patients need to be aware that not all information is the same, and that there is a lot of disinformation out there about prescription drugs, especially as concerns their efficacy and safety.

Today, blogs, discussion groups, social media sites, and others are inundated with personal opinions, without scrutiny or without including scientific reviews. For any ailment you will find websites that will also include which medications exist and how to use them. Such sources of information are rather to be considered as background noise, and you should always consult with your doctor or pharmacist about any concerns regarding prescribed or OTC (over the counter) drugs you are taking.

On the other hand, not all patients have the initiative to explore issues regarding their medications. Instead, they consider them to be *safe* if they are authorized for sale and prescribed by their doctors. Some patients rely absolutely on professional opinions, rarely question them, and sometimes not even fully understand why certain drugs are prescribed to them, nor how to use them.

Moreover, in my own family I had discussions regarding the use of over-the-counter medications like painkillers, marketed as 'the most recommended by doctors'. When I asked the question as of why would you take it, I got the answer ..."if it is over the counter and available for sale, it is safe and I can take as much of it as is recommended on the label....well, sometimes even more..." I was shocked with the answer and realized that people do not think as I do, and that, regardless of the fact that we, clinical research professionals, invest massive efforts in proving safety and efficacy of drugs that reach the market, the key safety information that we provide in the labelling does not transpire to the most important person, YOU!

I have thus come to realize that something had to be done; and that this 'something' should not be about pointing fingers, but rather about starting a conversation and creating solutions. Firstly, drug safety information should be available to all people in an easy and understandable language.

The informed patient is more compliant to treatment, and is less likely to suffer side effects caused by lack of understanding of the proper use of the prescribed drug and of the warning signs of its side effects.

Of course, it is important to remark that, as each of us is unique, we may react differently to drugs and therefore we may suffer a unique reaction not described anywhere, simply because it hasn't been previously observed. And that is unavoidable, as allergy to peanuts or seafood - it is an implied risk.

23

According to the CDC (Centers for Diseases Control and Prevention), every year there are approximately 123.8 million visits to the ER (emergency room) in the US, of which up to 38% are linked to reactions to medication. That is more than 47 million visits to the ER per year, all at a total cost of approximately 173 billion US dollars. Not to mention the pain and suffering that these situations may produce, while they are all   easy to avoid.

Chapter 1	Underlining important issues - Take away points
Issues	Not enough information on safety and effi-cacy of drugs is available in lay language
	Qualified information on the Internet is scarce.
	Blogs, discussion groups, social media may contain unreliable information.
Solutions	Empower patients through drug safety in-formation and education available to all people that is easy to read and understand

2

About drug development and how we got to where we are

Drugs, according to the FDA, are 'any product that is intended to be used to treat, prevent, diagnose or cure a disease'. Therefore, if we say that vitamin C cures scurvy, then it is considered a drug for regulatory purposes. That means that a product that contains vitamin C and is marketed for treating scurvy underwent rigorous scrutiny for its safety and efficacy including manufacturing procedures and quality.

Since the history of mankind, medicines have been studied and used to treat diseases, most of them from natural sources as herbal or animal extracts, minerals, concoctions, solutions, teas, ointments, and others.

Hippocrates and Galen, the great doctors of Ancient Greece, make extensive reference to the use of drugs in treating diseases. However, it was Paracelsus the first to understand the concept of dose and dosage. He pointed out that "any substance can be toxic and that it is the dose that differentiates the poison from the remedy". Also, nature cannot provide us with an unlimited source of pure active drugs that are cheap and easy enough to extract to make it *marketable* and *profitable*.

Developing and manufacturing a drug that can be stored for long periods of time, is limited when utilizing products from natural sources. The cost would be unaffordable, and in some cases, the shelf life is so extremely short that it makes no business sense to produce it at all.

We must also understand that drug research and development, as well as pharmaceutical manufacturing, is a *business*. Consequently, with the advent of industrialized chemical synthesis and mass production of chemicals, at the eve of the WWII, the pharmaceutical industry was shaped as a potential business powerhouse. The ability to mass produce small chemicals allowed pharmaceutical companies to develop and test millions of drugs that could potentially treat diseases. The market potential was enormous and the returns vast. But the regulators as the FDA had to evolve together with the industry in making sure that first and foremost the drugs are safe, and, since the late 1960's, also efficacious (meaning that they do work as intended).

Going back to the early 1900's, we have made great advances in drug therapies with penicillin first and then with sulphonamides to treat infections. A new world was opened with the treatment for infective diseases which until then were untreatable. These great discoveries were done at a time when clinical trials were rudimentary, and the approval process unsophisticated. Also, the first univalent[2] vaccines were developed in that period, which allowed to eradicate epidemics and crippling diseases. The industry progressed from chemical companies to large pharmaceutical hubs, initially in Europe and the US, and then all over the world.

However, in the 21st century the drug development process evolved as a very complex science, where from five thousands possible candidates of a new drug, only one may successfully get from discovery to the pharmacy. This success rate is small enough to discourage many investors.

---

[2]The word 'univalent' means that are intended to provide protection against only one microorganism.

The development process consists of several stages, starting from the *discovery* of a new chemical or biological entity of therapeutic interest. That entity has to be studied for potential toxicity and therapeutic use. Initially, we perform in vitro (in a test tube) and then in vivo (on animals) studies before we venture to expose the first human being to a research drug. That stage is called *pre-clinical development* and may take a few years, during which the majority of the products fail, mostly due to toxicity or lack of therapeutic interest. Once a potential product is identified as probably safe and has displayed some therapeutic potential in animals, it is tested on humans, starting with healthy volunteers (Phase I of Clinical Development). The rationale behind the use of healthy volunteers is to have the cleanest pharmacokinetic and safety data as possible without interference of diseases or other medications.

Although the rationale seems logical, there are lots of ethical concerns. Let us not forget that the subject on whom a new drug is tested, a healthy volunteer, does not benefit at all from the participation in these studies, while he or she assumes all the risks.

Further, if the product is deemed safe for healthy volunteers, meaning that the risk at taking the tested doses is acceptable, the product is developed (in the phases II and III) in patients who have the disease or condition the drug intends to treat. More than 80% of the study drugs fail before completing development due to many reasons, and one of which is SAFETY, more precisely put, where the *risk vs benefit ratio is not acceptable.*

In my expert opinion, the drug development process, as it exists in the present, is like shooting up blindfolded in the air with a large shotgun and waiting for a bird to fall. Sometimes we are lucky and a large duck is caught, and we have a blockbuster (like Viagra™) but most of the times the bullets are just lost, as are time, effort, and massive amounts of money.

Basically, discovering a new drug that can make a great advance in medicine by using the presently developed methods is almost like winning the lottery, but, if we do win, the windfall is astonishing. That is why pharmaceutical companies continue betting on potential drug candidates, if one succeeds, it is the jackpot!

So, here we are in the 21st century, utilizing a lot of resources and money and leaving it to a composite of luck and regulatory bodies' decisions, as they are the ones who decide what new drugs we can have available to treat health conditions in the future, including the newly identified diseases.

29

But we are getting further away from the topic I have the intention to discuss with you, and that is HAVE YOU EVER WONDERED IF YOUR PRESCRIPTION MEDICATION IS REALLY SAFE?

Chapter 2	Some history about drug development, and how we got to where we are - Take away points
FDA definition of drug	Any product that is intended to be used to treat, prevent, diagnose or cure a disease.
Therapeutic vs. toxic	Any substance can be toxic and it is the dose that differentiates the poison from the remedy.
Challenges of the pharmaceutical industry	Drug manufacturing has to be marketable and profitable. Drug research and development, as well as pharmaceutical manufacturing, is a business.
Drug development challenge	Drug development process evolved as a very complex science, where, from one thousand possible candidates of a new drug, only one may successfully get from discovery to the pharmacy. This success rate is small enough to discourage many investors.

3

A false sense of safety

The first thing I want to discuss is the concept of DRUG SAFETY before I embark on the discussion on how drugs can work safely.

The false sense of safety of either prescription or over-the-counter drugs comes from assuming in advance that, if they are sold in pharmacies, they must be safe.

Let's examine the following. The word safety, according to the latest edition of the Merriam Webster English dictionary is "the condition of being safe from undergoing or causing hurt, injury, or loss". Its synonym, the word security, means "freedom from danger".

Using common sense, we assume that if a drug is deemed safe by regulators, it means that it is free from danger, or we are safe from hurt, injury or loss.

Nevertheless, *it could not be farther from the truth!* Let me explain why.

What does it means when the FDA, or other regulatory agency for that matter, approves a drug for sale and says that it considers a drug safe for use in a particular group of patients, under prescribed conditions?

The answer is the following:

When the FDA or another health authority deems a drug safe for use in humans, it means that randomized controlled clinical trials (RCT) have been conducted on a selected sample of the patient population for the intended disease, and that it has been demonstrated that, under limited ideal conditions of treatment, the drug had a **favourable risk/ benefit ratio**.

So, what does it mean in plain language? It means that in RCTs the evidence shows that, **statistically, the benefit from taking the drug outweighs the risk from its side effects** or the risk from lack of treatment. Therefore, there are well documented risks, and those are very real.

Conversely, only drugs whose safety profile is deemed "acceptable" based on the data collected in clinical trials and later in post-marketing studies, in pharmacovigilance and in surveillance process, are the ones that we will reach the market and get prescribed.

Chapter 3	A false sense of safety - Take away points
The false sense of safety	Prescription or over-the-counter drugs are assumed in advance safe because they are sold in pharmacies.
Concept of DRUG SAFETY comes from extrapolating definitions	The dictionary definition of the word SAFE means "The condition of being safe from undergoing or causing hurt, injury, or loss". Its synonym, the word security, means "freedom from danger. Hence we assume that if a drug is deemed safe by regulators, it means that is free from danger, or that we are safe from hurt, injury or loss. This is not true in the context of drug safety.
What does the FDA or other agency mean when they approve a drug?	It means that randomized controlled clinical trials (RCT) have been conducted on a selected sample of the patient population for the intended disease, and that it was demonstrated that, under limited ideal conditions of treatment, the drug had a favourable risk/benefit ratio.
A drug is safe when…	In RCTs the evidence shows that statistically the benefit from taking the drug outweighs the risk from its side effects or the risk from lack of treatment.

Chapter 3	A false sense of safety - Take away points (continuation)
Which drugs are going to reach the market and then prescribed?	Only those drugs whose safety profile is deemed "acceptable" based on the data collected in clinical trials and later in post-marketing studies, in pharma-covigilance and in the surveillance process.

4

Acceptable risk/benefit ratio is what it's all about

The next logical question is how the criteria for acceptability are developed. This is an issue where we can enumerate many philosophical stances, opinions and positions. But the most honest answer would be that "*it depends*".

The acceptability of a drug safety profile may depend on the disease that we intend to treat. For example, if the disease is very serious and the patient can die from it, a potential drug that may save or extend the patient's life is permitted to potentially present more side effects and more risks than a drug we would use to treat a minor condition, in which case only mild and minimum side effects will be acceptable.

The acceptability of the safety profile of a drug is based on expert opinions of leading scientists and medical experts on the condition the drug intends to treat. That opinion may be greatly influenced by a countless number factors as is for instance the availability of any other drug on the market to treat that same condition, or the profile of patients who may benefit from it, or how much data is provided to support the safety.

There is no global consensus on how the acceptability of risk and benefits is assessed and quantified; hence, there will be some drugs approved in the EU that are not approved in the US and vice versa.

Having defined safety of a drug as a favourable ratio between its risk and its benefit, I have to elaborate now on the concept of **risk,** from the perspective of a therapeutic product, and also its **benefit**.

Risk is defined as the possibility of loss or injury. In the case of drug therapy, both loss and injury are part of the equation of risk. In the pharmaceutical industry, when a drug is marketed there are many parties assuming risks, the one with the biggest stakes being the patient, as it is the patient that risks his/her own life.

There is also the risk is assumed by the company manufacturing and selling the product. It is mainly the financial risk of liability for injuries potentially caused by the side effects of a drug (whether they were described in the labelling information or not). Therefore, we tend to favour drugs that bear less risk not only because we want to keep patients safe but because we want to preserve companies from liability.

There are many parties assuming risks when a prescription drug is dispensed. Risks are also assumed by insurers, health care providers and health care facilities, as well as the manufacturers, and we must also not exclude the risk the drug potentially poses to the environment (either from metabolites or by-products released in the environment after use in the manufacturing process, or when discarded).

The risk equation of a drug product cannot be a standardized formula, neither can it be expressed numerically, and is basically assumed and concluded from favorable and non-favorable opinions by experts who may or may not have declared conflicts of interest[3] on the particular product.

---

[3] Declared conflict of interest implies that the experts are paid or receive monies in lieu of shares or investment from the same company they are reviewing the drug product for.

41

Mainly, the assessment of risk consists of evidence gathered in pre-clinical and clinical development in a sample that is not necessarily a statistically random sample, but represents a number of subjects selected according to criteria mainly dictated by the outcome that is sought. Therefore, risk is assessed in what I call a "biased sample" of a limited number of subjects that often present a pretty much similar set of characteristics.

To make myself clear, let me represent the population that has a particular disease that we intend to enrol in a study, on the pie chart in the figure 1.

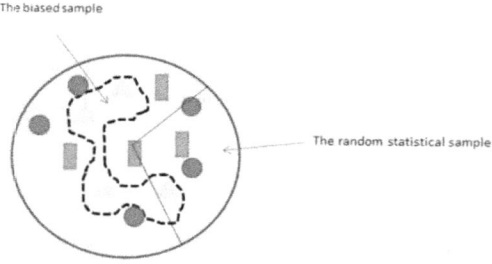

Figure 1 – Simple representation of patient population with hypertension. The circles represent patients with hypertension and diabetes; the squares represent the patients with hypertension and previous myocardial infarction, and the triangles represent patients that are moderately hypertensive, but otherwise healthy. The dotted line is the sample in a clinical trial.

The slice on this pie would represent a random statistical sample for test and analysis in clinical trials. However, that is not the case in clinical research. In clinical trials, the protocol dictates who can be part of a study. We will pick and choose the subjects in order to *reduce risk* and *achieve development goals*. In this case, we want to try an antihypertensive drug. So I choose patients who do not have any diagnosed underlying condition but only hypertension, and thus purposely exclude others with previous myocardial infarction or diabetes, theoretically disregarding that those excluded might represent the real market the drug attains. That is what I call a ***biased sample***. All safety and efficacy data, as well as the risk assessment, are performed on a biased sample. Consequently, we do not have the information on how the drug may behave in the real world. This is what I call *"**the drug development fallacy**"*. We assume that, when you take the prescription medication, there will be a good probability that the drug behaves as observed in randomized clinical trials with the ideally selected patients treated under controlled strict procedures. But, it may not…

The drug gets approved only if it fulfills a pre-established set of safety and efficacy as well as quality requirements, after which marketing takes over to guarantee the best returns on the investment in the shortest period of time. I must not forget to mention one key factor in the race for market success, mainly, very early in development, once a drug is identified as being of interest, it is patented. For 20 years, the pharmaceutical company is protected from the generic competition. In that period of time, they have to develop the drug, run clinical trials, and submit it to regulatory authorities for approval, which may take a whopping 12 or more years on average, costing about 2 billion dollars as per 2013 average projection per drug.

After that, if the drug gets approved by the regulators, the manufacturers have to make enough money to return the 2 billion USD invested in its development. Further, it has to generate good revenues for the shareholders who waited patiently for those 12 years, after having invested those 2 billion USD with the probability of losing being more than in 80%.

However, let's go back to acceptable risk vs. benefit assessment.

Just recently, the regulators came up with a strategy to minimize the effect of the aforementioned fallacy in drug development, through the development of a Risk Evaluation and Mitigation Strategy (REMS) in the US-FDA, which also

44

exists in a different modality in Europe and Canada as of lately. With this strategy, pharmaceutical companies are obliged by regulation to continue studying the drug well into post-marketing (once the drug is available for sale) period, to collect real world data, with the aim to verify whether clinical trial data were concurrent to the one obtained with the sample population originally exposed to the drug, or if the effect of the drug turned out to be different. In the latter case, a new risk/benefit reassessment has to be done to ensure continuity of the marketability of the product. In brief, the clinical trial will continue well into the marketing phase, and that is just because we either were not be able to observe all the possible risks and effects of a drugs in the years of development, or because the clinical trials did not include certain underrepresented population. This strategy is aimed at capturing safety information which was not made available during clinical development due to a number of reasons including the limitation on the exposure of the drug to patients, or limited time. This means that development costs will go drastically up in the future, and that pharmaceutical companies will not be able to reduce the price of the product when it establishes itself in the market. Note that generic companies do not have any responsibility whatsoever to study the safety or efficacy of the products they manufacture in clinical trials. They solely rely on the data already captured by the brand name companies when the product was developed and are required limited bioequivalence studies.

In summary, DRUG SAFETY refers to a perception of risk and benefit in function of many variables that depend on the nature of the disease and the outcome expected, as well as on potential liabilities.

When a drug is deemed safe for human use, this only refers to the limited knowledge based on RTC (randomized controlled clinical trials) conducted on a specific patient population, under very limited and controlled circumstances, and do not intend to portray otherwise.

The RISK for the patient arising from drug treatment, is based on the assumption that loss or injury can occur regardless of the precautions taken and data accrued, and that risk, as such, is inherent to any human activity. The key here is whether the level of risk is acceptable enough to meet the challenge.

Chapter 4	Acceptable risk/benefit ratio is what it's all about - Take away points
Criteria for acceptability for the risk-benefit ratio	Depends on many factors as for instance the disease to be treated (the more serious condition, the more risky drugs are allowed. i.e. chemotherapeutic agents in cancer therapy).
What is the acceptability of the safety profile based on?	The acceptability of the safety profile of a drug is based on, 1. Expert opinions of leading scientists and medical experts on the condition the drug intends to treat. 2. That opinion may be greatly influenced by a countless number of factors as is for instance **a**. the availability of any other drug on the market to treat that same condition, or **b**. the profile of patients who may benefit from it, or how much data is provided to support the safety.
Why are drugs approved in one country and not in another?	There is no global consensus on how the acceptability of risk and benefits is assessed and quantified; hence, there will be some drugs approved in the EU that are not approved in the US and vice versa.
What does 'risk' mean?	Risk is defined as the possibility of loss or injury. In the case of drug therapy, both loss and injury are part of the equation of risk.

Chapter 4	Acceptable risk/benefit ratio is what it's all about - Take away points (continuation)
Who assumes the risk?	The company manufacturing and selling the product. Risks are also assumed by insurers, health care providers and health care facilities, as well as the manufacturers, and we must also not exclude the risk the drug potentially poses to the environment (either from metabolites or by-products released in the environment after use in the manufacturing process, or when discarded). The ones with the biggest stakes are the patients, as they risk their own health and life.
How is risk calculated?	The risk equation cannot be a standardized formula, neither can it be expressed numerically, and is basically assumed and concluded from favorable and non-favorable opinions by experts who may or may not have declared conflicts of interest on the particular product.
What is the drug development fallacy?	The statistical sample that is used for clinical trials does not represent the actual population with a particular disease, but is a carefully selected sample of individuals with limited conditions and characteristics that are all similar.

Chapter 4	Acceptable risk/benefit ratio is what it's all about - Take away points (continuation)
What is the drug development fallacy? (continuation)	We will pick and choose the subjects for a clinical trial in order to reduce risk and achieve goals. Therefore, I consider that a biased sample. Doctors assume that the data provided in the specifications of prescription drugs correspond to a statistical sample free from bias and therefore they can extrapolate and assume the response on their individual patients.
Why time of development is of essence?	Patents provide protection for 20 years. There, companies have to develop the drug, run clinical trials, and submit it to regulators for approval, which may take 12 or more years on average, costing about 2 billion dollars as per 2013 average per drug.
How to reduce the effect of the drug development fallacy?	Regulators developed a strategy to reduce the effect of the fallacy in drug development, with a Risk Evaluation and Mitigation Strategy (REMS) in the US-FDA. In REMS, companies have to continue studying the drug well into post-marketing period, to collect real world data, with the aim to verify whether clinical trial data were concurrent to the one obtained with the sample population originally exposed to the drug, or if the effect of the drug is different.

Chapter 4	Acceptable risk/benefit ratio is what it's all about - Take away points (continuation)
End objective of REMS	Capturing safety information which was not made available during clinical development due to a number of reasons including the limitation on the exposure of patients to the drug, or limited time.
What about generic companies?	Generic companies do not have any responsibility whatsoever to study the safety or efficacy of the products they manufacture in clinical trials. They solely rely on the data already captured by the brand name companies when the product was developed and are required a limited number of bioequivalence studies.
What does DRUG SAFETY mean?	DRUG SAFETY refers to a perception of risk and benefit in function of many variables that depend on the nature of the disease and the outcome expected, as well as on potential liabilities.
What does it means that a drug is safe in humans?	This only refers to the limited knowledge based on RTC (randomized controlled clinical trials) conducted on a specific patient population, under very limited and controlled circumstances, and do not intend to portray otherwise.
What does drug treatment risk mean for a patient?	It is based on the assumption that loss or injury can occur regardless of the precautions taken and data accrued, and that risk, as such, is inherent to any human activity. The key here is whether the level of risk is acceptable enough to meet the challenge.

5

In addition to being safe, drugs have to provide a benefit

The perceived benefit of a therapeutic product is based on many assumptions, including the fact that we suppose that each potential patient who is prescribed a particular drug will have an average response to it, that the patient is of average size, built, and age, and also that gender differences are not always a factor for differential prescription.

The benefit of a drug depends on the ability of the therapeutic product to improve the particular condition it intends to treat when compared to taking no treatment at all, taking placebo or other less efficacious standard treatments. That benefit has to be clinically significant, meaning the improvement is not marginal but good enough to be worth the risk.

It is important to highlight here that the majority of drugs seldom *cure* a condition, with the exception of some, like antibiotics. Drugs in general only reduce or control certain symptoms enough to allow the body to pull through, to permit life routine, and to continue the best possible, as is the case with a pain reliever; or to control certain abnormality as is with insulin that is designed to normalize blood sugar or with statins that lower cholesterol level.

One of the biggest misconceptions that the average patient has about medications is that a medication will cure all their ailments. That cannot be farther from the truth.

To make certain ideas clear, let me classify drugs according to their expected therapeutic benefits, and thus allow the reader to understand the potential expectations the patients may have when they are prescribed a medication.

I divided all therapeutic products into seven categories according to the expected therapeutic benefits, for illustration purposes. These categories do not always imply classification according to a specific disease. These are drugs that serve to either prevent a disease, to control symptoms or a condition, to reverse a condition, life-savings drugs, to cure a disease, and the recent category of life-style medications.

The first category includes drugs *intended to prevent a disease,* and the best example of that are vaccines. Vaccines allowed the eradication of polio, and other crippling diseases improving extensively children as well as adult survival, health and quality of life. See table 1-Drug categories according to the expected therapeutic benefit.

The second category encompasses drugs aimed at *controlling symptoms* or a medical condition. The vast majority of drugs presently prescribed fall under this category. They are used, for example, to control blood sugar, pressure and cholesterol, pain, anxiety, epilepsy, and the progression of other diseases. In general, they are intended to be used for life, creating issues concerning very long term safety and accumulation. Very long term safety data cannot be obtained through clinical trials, since it is impossible to follow subjects for very long periods of time due to the modalities of drug development processes, timeliness and cost.

Presently, with post-marketing and registry[4] studies, the pharmaceutical industry and regulators aim at addressing very long term safety and efficacy, i.e. what is called 'efficiency' in the real world.

Table 1 - Drug categories according to the expected therapeutic benefit	
1	Prevent a disease
2	Control symptoms
3	Reverse a condition
4	Life saving
5	Cure a disease
6	Life-style medications
7	Diagnose diseases or conditions

---

[4] Registry studies are aimed at collecting data from actual patients in the clinic setting to compare different medical interventions and their outcomes.

The third category consists of ***drugs used to reverse symptoms*** or a condition. These drugs intend to replace an either deficient or non-existent but necessary hormone or other endogenous (produced by the own body) substance necessary for the normal body function. This category of drugs are very limited, mostly biologics[5], and although they do not comprise a large market, are very commonly used. These drugs have their own category because they are able to re-establish the normal functioning of the body with established side effects, but if we discontinue the treatment, the condition reappears as originally diagnosed. For example, clotting factors in hemophilia, or levothyroxine in hypothyroidism, belong to this group.

The fourth category is ***lifesaving drugs***. These drugs are generally used in an emergency situation to save a patient's life, as epinephrine, or even saline solution to rehydrate a patient. Also, the commonly known EpiPen™, which is continuously carried by people who are at risk to develop anaphylaxis. These drugs fall under a wide spectrum of chemical entities, but are nevertheless used to save a patient's life. These drugs are extremely important, and are normally used only

---

[5] Biologics are drugs developed with the use of recombinant DNA technology to produce proteins with therapeutic intent

once or a couple of times in the emergency situation, until the patient is stabilized.

The fifth category is the drugs *that cure a condition or a disease*. We wish that all drugs could cure, but *they do not*. However, some drugs do, as are antibiotics and anti-parasitic drugs. These drugs revolutionized medicine, and allowed people to live without the morbidity of a chronic infection. Tuberculosis, stomach ulcers, ear and throat infections, for instance, have become temporary conditions that can be effectively cured with this category of drugs. Although resistance to antibiotics has been developed, new molecules are being studied to avoid the reappearance of infections that can be life-threatening or even kill a person.

The sixth category that I will discuss here are *life-style medications*. These prescribed medications are utilized to improve performance in various areas of life when prescribed to otherwise healthy people. Birth control medication falls under this category, and erectile dysfunction drugs used not for the purpose of treating a disease, but enhancing performance.

The last category is drugs used to *diagnose diseases or conditions* as are contrasting agents in computer tomography scans (CT-scans). See table 2- Drug categories and examples.

Table 2	Classification of therapeutic products according to expected therapeutic benefit		
Drug desired effect	Examples in General Terms	Examples in Generic Terms	Beneficial characteristics
Prevention of a disease	Vaccines	Polio, flu, small pox, whopping cough vaccines	This therapeutic product prevents the disease and condition, avoiding epidemics. Children may benefit the most.
Control of a condition or symptom	Anti-hypertensive (drugs to control blood pressure)	Diuretics, beta blockers, ACE inhibitors, calcium channel blockers, etc	These drugs do not cure hypertension, but controls blood pressure utilizing different bimolecular mechanisms

Table 2	Classification of therapeutic products according to expected therapeutic benefit (continuation)		
Control of a condition or symptom	Hypo-glycemic (drugs to control blood sugar)	Sulfonylureas, metformin, glinides, alpha glycosidase inhibitors, insulin, etc.	These drugs do not cure diabetes, but control blood sugar to avoid or delay the effects of the disease
	Anti-histaminic (drugs to control allergic reactions)	Dexamethasone fexofenadine, diphenhydramine, loratadine, brompheniramine, cetirizine, etc.	These drugs reduce the effects of allergies inhibiting the release of histamine
	Anti-arrhythmic (to control heart rhythm)	Beta blockers, antiplatelet agents	These drugs controls the symptoms of arrhythmia

Table 2	Classification of therapeutic products according to expected therapeutic benefit (continuation)		
Reverse a condition	Hormone replacement therapy	Estrogen, progesterone, levothyroxine	The effects of these drugs are temporary and only present when the drug is taken.
	Blood clotting factors	Factor VIII or Factor IX, desmopressin	
Life-saving drugs	Any drug utilized in emergency setting to save a patient life	Physiological saline solution (I.V.), streptoki-nase, aspirin, adrenaline,	These drugs when used in an emergency setting may save the life of a patient
	Antibiotics, anti-parasitic agents	Penicillin, azithromycin, amoxicillin, norfloxacin, etc.	These drugs kill or inhibit the growth of the pathogen and hence cure

Table 2	Classification of therapeutic products according to expected therapeutic benefit (continuation)		
Life-style drugs	Erectile dysfunction drugs used in healthy males, oral contraceptives	Tadalafil, sildenafil, varden-afil, Levonorg-estrel/ethinyl estradiol, Desoges-trel/ethinyl estradiol	These drugs have a temporary effect on a normal body function. Note that I included erectile dysfunction drugs in this section since despite the condition to be treated, is because is utilizes when intercourse is sough hence not particularly necessary for daily activities.
Diagnose a disease or condition	Contrasting agents for CT scans MRI's and x-rays	Gadolinium, barium, io-dine, radioi-sotopes,	Utilized to enhance the contrast in diagnostic imaging to make it possible to see abnormalities

Chapter 5	In addition to being safe, drugs have to provide a benefit - Take away points
What is the expected benefit from drug therapy?	The perceived benefit is based on many assumptions, including the fact that we suppose that each potential patient who is prescribed a particular drug will have an average response to it that the patient is of average size, built, age, and also that gender differences are not always a factor for differential prescription.
What does the benefit of a drug therapy depend on?	The benefit of a drug depends on the ability of the therapeutic product to improve the particular condition it intends to treat when compared to taking no treatment at all, taking placebo or other less efficacious standard treatments.
Which are the main beneficial drug effects?	Prevent a disease, Control symptoms, Reverse a condition, Life-saving, Cure disease .Lifestyle medications. Also drugs are used for diagnostic purposes

6

One size does not fit all, the tale of *personalized medicine*

You may have heard of the concept of *personalized medicine* as the new approach to therapeutic interventions.

Pharmaceutical companies as well as regulators are investing great amount of resources and efforts in developing treatments tailored to individual patients' needs. The future of medicine is heading towards personalization.

You may be asking yourself why?

In order to understand the change in the approach to developing therapeutic products, it is important to know where it all came from.

In the past, when a therapeutic product was being developed, in order to make it marketable, pharmaceutical companies would select those drug candidates that could be prescribed to most of the patients with a particular condition. The idea was that a new chemical or biological entity, which was to improve a certain symptom, would have to make both clinical and economic sense. Also, the favoured dosage form is what I call 'the magic pill', figuratively speaking, or 'solid oral forms'[6].

In the past, pharmacology assumed that all patients would respond in the same manner to a drug product, and that potential differences in the way the drug worked were not clinically relevant. Hence, safety was the most important characteristic of a drug that a company had to prove to obtain market approval. The concept started to lose significance with the introduction of evidence-based medicine and randomized controlled clinical trials (RCT), which have made potential differences in the way a drug works become very relevant.

Characteristics like age, gender, race, underlying conditions (other diseases the patient may have), concomitant medications (other drugs the patient may be taking), weight and body mass index, smoking, drinking and eating habits, geographical location and, most recently, genetic makeup, proved to be very relevant in terms of drug re-

---

[6] Pill that is taken by mouth

sponse. We observed that, pharmacologically speaking, reactions to the same drug were different enough between individuals to be notable.

We started observing that there were groups of people that responded very well to a drug (it means that the drug achieved control over the symptom as expected) and tolerated the drug well. On the other hand, there were other groups that proved more sensitive to the drug and developed adverse drug reactions (side effects) unique to that group of people. Others yet did not respond at all, while just a few developed catastrophic adverse drug reactions (life threatening or even death). Observing similar results across clinical trials with different drugs and in different indications, made us think that even when belonging to a more or less homogeneous group according to measurable external characteristics, patients were pharmacologically different.

Randomized controlled clinical trials demonstrated that we were not only different in the way we respond to treatment, but had different sensitivities which required more attention.

Those differences, once identified, increased the degree of uncertainty regarding how a new therapeutic product would be positioned in the market, since until recently the axiom of the drug industry was that "one size fits all". If a product did not fit the needs of most of the patients within a population for a particular disease, it meant that the company would lose market share for that condition and producing that particular drug would not make business sense.

Let's see an example in order to have a clearer idea of how drug products are developed, from the point of view of the active ingredient, dosage form (type of pill or capsule, for instance) and strength (amount of active drug in a pill).

Assume that a shoe manufacturer decides to maximize their profits and makes only shoes size 11. The marketing strategy would be that everyone (male, female, children, elderly, etc.) who has at least one foot could wear and enjoy them, and that the shoe will protect people from the dirt on the floor surface. Let's assume now that a young woman buys the shoes, but her foot size is 7. She would be able to put them very comfortably on her feet, but walking will be difficult since they are too big. Nevertheless, the foot is protected. Then we have an adult man buying the shoes, and he is a size 11, therefore he leaves the store very happy and does not have any inconvenience. However, we may have an elderly female, who is size 8 and she also buys the shoes that are size 11. She has similar problems as the young woman has and in addition she falls and breaks her hip because the shoe was too loose. This example is ideal to illustrate how the pharmaceutical industry considers that there is an optimal dose that can be applied to all patients for most of the drugs developed (with some exceptions), and that if a patient takes an average dose, he/she would have an average response that would make clinical sense. In this case, wearing the size 11 shoe will allow the subject to have the feet protected (equivalent to the concept to drug efficacy) but some people will have problems walking due to the size that is too big or too small (equivalent to side effects that are not too serious, similar to the difficulty in walking because the shoe is too big). But other side effects can be catastrophic, equivalent to the old woman in the shoe metaphor who falls and breaks her hip.

This early approach allowed for the production of only few dose strengths (sometimes only a scored tablet in order to allow the patient to break it in half), which reduced the product development and manufacturing costs enormously and increased revenues prodigiously. However, once RTC (randomized controlled clinical trials) become the gold standard to demonstrate safety and efficacy of new drugs, the resulting data started to show that there are subpopulations (small groups of patients) that responded favorably, while other people did not responded partially or not at all, or, worse yet, some were more prone to serious side effects. That is how the RTC has demonstrated that one size does not fit all, and the old axiom of the pharmaceutical product development ceased to exist.

The differences observed on drug response in a population reside in their genes. Our genetic make-up plays a key role in our health and in our potential to develop diseases. Also, our genes dictate how we are going to respond to medications.

With advances in genetic sequencing technology, we were able to identify minute variations in our genetic code that dictate if we are going to respond well to a drug, or have unusual sensibilities. Those minute variations are called SNPs (snips, or single nucleotide polymorphisms). The ability to identify those SNPs allowed us to understand the variability in drug response and sensitivities in different people in the same population group. That new area in pharmacology that allows us to identify SNPs in patients is called pharmacogenomics and the test is called pharmacogenomics test (PGx test). Nevertheless, the PGx test limits the use of drugs the way they used to be in the past, where with the trial and error method doctors were able to determine the best therapy and ascertain the optimal dose. PGx-DNA testing allows us to identify those polymorphisms and recognize patients who should take certain type of drugs to control their symptoms, and thus determine to which active ingredient they will respond best so as to also reduce the risk of suffering serious side effects.

In short that is what *"personalized medicine* is all about".

Before you obtain your next prescription, you may or may not be tested for SNPs to determine the most appropriate therapy. It is most likely that you will not, since access to these tests is very limited and expensive, it is not included in the requirement for prescription, or the tests are simply unavailable to general public but only in clinical trials or in a limited fashion.

Chapter 6	One size does not fit all, the tale of personalized medicine- Take away points
Personalized medicine	Focuses on developing therapies tailored to patients' needs.
The past of pharmaceutical development	Pharmaceutical companies would select those drug candidates that could be prescribed to most of the patients with a particular condition, in order to make it marketable. Pharmacology assumed that all patients would respond in the same manner, and that potential differences were not clinically relevant.
Dosage form selected	Depends, the favoured dosage form is the 'solid oral forms'.
The present of pharmaceutical development	Evidence-based medicine and randomized controlled clinical trials (RCT), to detect potential differences in the way a drug works in different patients.
The old axiom of pharmaceutical development	Until recently the axiom of the drug industry was that "one size fits all", therefore all patients got the same dose. This early approach allowed for the production of only few dose strengths (sometimes only a scored tablet in order to allow the patient to break it in half).

Chapter 6	One size does not fit all, the tale of personalized medicine- Take away points
Why are there differences in drug responses?	The differences observed in drug response in a population reside in the patients genes. Minute variations in our genetic code response. Those minute variations are called SNPs.
What SNPs have to do with drug therapy?	The ability to identify those SNPs allowed us to understand the variability in drug response and sensitivities in different people in the same population group. That new area in pharmacology that allows us to identify SNPs in patients is called pharmacogenomics and the test is called pharmacogenomics test (PGx test).
The PGx test	PGx-DNA testing allows us to identify those polymorphisms and recognize patients who should take certain type of drugs to control their symptoms, and thus determine to which active ingredient they will respond best so as to also reduce the risk of suffering serious side effects.

7

Why your prescription drug is not working anymore?

The answer to the question of why your prescription drug is not working anymore is not simple. There are many factors that may be influencing your lack of response to a prescription drug you have been taking for a long time and were used to it. **(NOTE-you should always consult with your doctor or pharmacist if you consider that the prescription drug you are taking is not working anymore).**

One reason may be that you have developed *tolerance.* That means that, in the course of time, your body got used to the drug in such way that the drug cannot control your symptoms anymore. This can be easily determined if you are still using the same bottle that you used to respond well to and suddenly you stopped responding.

However, if you were dispensed a new lot of the same drug, in the same strength, many other things may happen. Let's look at different scenarios.

Firstly, you should check if the prescription dispensed is the same as before. Dispensing errors might occur and they are very dangerous. What you should check is if the drug looks the same, is from the same manufacturer and if it is the same dosage strength as before.

If in doubt, you can consult a pill identifier website[7]. That web site will tell you not only if the drug you were dispensed is the one that was prescribed to you, but will also show you the shape, color, size, imprint, and who the manufacturer is. You can also find further details there about the drug you are taking.

If the drug corresponds to the one you were prescribed and is from the same manufacturer and in the same dosage strength as before but the therapeutic effect has changed,

---

[7] For example
http://www.drugs.com/pill_identification.html

- you might have developed some tolerance to it, or
- you may not have the very same type of condition and you may need another drug, or,
- you may have been added a new drug and it interferes with this one, producing an unwanted drug interaction, or
- there might have been a problem with the batch of your prescription and you may need to refill with a new one.

Regardless, always consult your doctor or health provider when your drug is not working.

Another potential issue arises when the prescription you are given is for the same drug and dosage strength, but by a different manufacturer. In that case, you might experience problems due to the fact that generic drugs are only bioequivalent to the brand name you used to have, and, when getting dispensed another brand of generic, the pharmaceutical equivalence may not be there, and you either need a dose adjustment or to go back to your original brand.

Regardless of these explanations, again, you must consult your doctor or pharmacist without delay if you suspect that your drug is not working anymore. If you fail to do so, your condition (e.g. diabetes, hypertension, arrhythmia, depression, anxiety, paranoia, etc.) may go untreated and that may momentarily lead to even more serious problems.

Chapter 7	Why your prescription drug is not working anymore - Take away points
Factors influencing drug response	Tolerance, dispensing errors, development of a new disease or condition, drug or supplements interactions, generic not pharmaceutically equivalent.

8

How can you know if the side effects are expected

Drugs have many effects besides the desired one, i.e. the benefit we are looking for. The reason for this is because the drug is a molecule that generally binds (sticks) to receptors on cells of many different tissues in the body. We can predict effects of a drug based on its ability to distribute though the body. In order to be able to market a new drug, pharmaceutical companies have to determine which is the most beneficial therapeutic effect and the optimal dose to achieve it. However, the drug may have effects on all other cells, not only the ones we want to treat, and at different levels. Such effects that a patient may experience at therapeutic doses are called *side effects*.

After the previous explanation, you realize that we can always expect a certain degree of side effects. The key here is that they must be minimal and reversible (it means that they disappear with the discontinuation of the drug).

This is why we conduct studies for safety and tolerability of drugs before making them available in the market. Following the successful completion of the said studies, we can assume that drugs at the established doses are TOLERABLE, meaning that any side effect should be reversible and not toxic. For instance, if you start taking an antibiotic, the expected side effect is diarrhea, and that is because the drug started working and killing all microorganisms, including the good ones in your gut. That side effect may become serious to such an extent that the diarrhea makes you dehydrate and you can end-up in ER with an intra-venous solution hooked up (which should rarely occur), or they can be minimal, in which case they disappear within a few day (preferred in the safety profile of the drug).

In summary, you can always expect some kind of side effects, they are part of the effects of the drug, they may be minimal and benign, or very serious or life-threatening. Normally, only drugs that have minimal and non-life-threatening side effects that have been observed in a limited population during clinical trials are allowed on the market. Nonetheless, some people may have specific susceptibility to a drug or one of its components, like allergy, or develop other severe reactions due to their genetic makeup. Those are impossible to foresee, therefore all drugs should be taken with caution, since each patient is unique and each patient is a "clinical trial" apart.

Another side effect that is worth discussing here again, is *lack of efficacy*. Some people do not respond to the prescribed drugs as expected, and that can be very serious, especially in conditions that are severe or life threatening (hypertension, arrhythmia, anaphylaxis, etc.). You may not respond to a medication because of your particularities, hence a change in your prescription will be necessary to control your condition. Always consult your doctor when you suspect that your medication does not work.

Chapter 8	How can you know if the side effects are expected - Take away points
What are side effects?	They are part of the effects of the drug, they may be minimal and benign, or very serious or life threatening. Normally, only drugs that have mini-mal and non-life-threatening side effects that have been observed in a limited popula-tion during clinical trials are allowed on the market. Side effects are all unwanted effects that a drug may have at therapeutic dos-es. They should be minimal and reversible
Tolerability of a drug	When the side effects at the thera-peutic doses are bearable within certain parameters of safety.
Can I expect side effects?	You can always expect some kind of side effects, they are part of the effects of the drug, they may be minimal and benign, or very seri-ous or life threaten-ing. You must be aware of the side effects to expect, and when to contact the doctor or pharmacist.
Is lack of efficacy a side effect?	Yes, some people do not respond to the prescribed drugs as ex-pected, and that can be very seri-ous, especially in conditions that are severe or life threatening.

9

Should you influence your doctor's decision on which drug to prescribe you?

In general, doctors prescribe the best option that is available for the type of condition you have, taking into account your overall health, other medication you may be taking, and your insurance coverage, of course. Before writing the prescription, your doctor may ask you about your co-pay or the type of coverage for prescription medications if relevant, or he/she may recommend an option that may not be covered but is the best for you.

If you live in the United States, you are exposed to information on prescription drugs and their characteristics on a daily basis, through TV ads, billboards and printed magazines, as well as the

Internet, Although the law permits this in the United States, when drug manufacturers are targeting you with that information, that means they are indirectly encouraging you to "ask your doctor" for it. On the one hand, the information provided in that advertising material has been approved by the FDA and presents the prescription drug in light of the information the *reasonable patient* would like and should know. On the other hand, we have the vast majority of countries where it is strictly prohibited to advertise prescription medication directly to patients, since it is considered that the patient is not the one who should be making the choice, but rather to go through a prescribing physician who is going to prescribe the drug and therefore be the main decision-maker since he/she is qualified to do so. In some countries, not all physicians can prescribe all medications. Rather, only selected specialists can prescribe certain type of medications, as for instance anti-depressants. There are different approaches to marketing prescription drugs, and although it is not the aim of this book to discuss drug marketing policies, I will give you my opinion on the matter, in the context of whether you should be influencing your doctor's decision or not.

You may be an engineer by profession, an architect, cook, housewife, teacher, journalist, etc. Your education prepared you for your work. Just as I do

not know what is needed to build a house or pro-
gram a computer, your ability as an educated
person, regardless of your level of education or
experience, is to perform the job you were prepared to do at the best of your ability. You may
have had some courses of biology and chemistry
in your life. Nevertheless, with all due respect for
your education, that education does not prepare
you to diagnose your disease or assume that you
can decide on which type of drugs you should be
prescribed.

If you saw a new drug to control blood pressure
in an ad, or if you saw your friend taking a new
drug and you want it too, it does not make you
qualified to make the decision to take it. Therapeu-
tics is a branch of pharmacology that focuses on
the way drugs are prescribed. Your doctor is
expected to be highly trained in it, so he/she
should decide what the best option for your treatment is.

Having said that, I also affirm that it is your ob-
ligation as a patient to educate yourself in what
your disease or condition is, how you can improve
your habits to feel better, and, if needed, which
medication you should take and how to avoid
further deterioration of your health. *As a patient,
you should be part of the decision,* while taking
into account the information your doctor provided,

the information your pharmacists gave you, as well as the truthful information gathered elsewhere.

Prescription drugs, as well as over-the-counter medication, or even certain foods and drinks, can have serious impact on your health and wellbeing. The right dose and type of medication can make a great difference. Remember that prescription drugs are not free from unwanted effects, and you should always know about them, so as to be able to react fast if there is a problem, since your doctor is not there 24/7 to see how you react to a drug.

On the other hand, it may happen that your condition is not properly controlled by the medication you are prescribed and you may experience side effects that are very bothersome. In that case, you should go back to your doctor and see if there is a better option for you. You may do some research yourself, and get familiar with the medications that can help you. There may even be a new drug in the market that you are willing to try since you do not feel better with what you are presently taking. Remember, your health is your responsibility. Make a list of questions you want to ask your doctor during the next visit. I advise you to ask as many questions as you can. You should write the answers down if you need to remember important things, but do not challenge the doctors' knowledge. Do not be a "wiki-patient[8]". Be *patient* and polite, and if you disagree, go elsewhere for a second opinion. Some doctors are comfortable prescribing a certain set of drugs, but do not feel easy prescribing a brand new drug until more clinical experience is gathered.

Although you can ask if there is a better option for you, you should **not request** for a specific drug, especially if your doctor does not believe that it is the best and safest option. Your doctor is liable for your prescription, and he/she will write it to the best of their ability.

On the other hand, there are two scenarios that I personally believe you should be firm about when asking for a specific medication.

The first one is, you are comfortable with your medication, it controls your symptoms well and you do not have bothersome side effects, but your doctor wants to change your prescription to a new one. You should ask to continue with the drug that is already working for you, unless the reason for the change is because the drug is either in shortage or it was determined that is not safe anymore and

---

[8] Wiki-patient is a patient that browsed the condition or the drug on the internet and challenges the doctors knowledge with information that may not be properly qualified

there is evidence that it can seriously harm you in the long run.

The other scenario is, if you were on the brand name of the product (called the originator drug) and your doctor is changing you to the generic alternative because it is cheaper or because the insurance will only pay for the cheapest generic alternative. In that case, if you feel uncomfortable with the change, be firm and pay for the difference. Sometimes you may not have the choice since the originator drug is no longer available. Then you will have to discuss that situation with your doctor and make a decision whether to continue with the generic alternative or to try a new drug.

Always ask your doctor before making any decision about your prescription drugs.

Never discontinue a drug unless you have a serious reaction, in which case you should go to your nearest ER.

Do not feel shy or intimidated by your doctor. Ask questions, you have the right to be informed, and it is also your responsibility to care for your own health.

Chapter 9	Should you influence your doctor's decision on which drug to prescribe you?- Take away points
The role of prescription drug marketing	In the US, it is allowed to market directly to patients including marketing information approved by the FDA. In other countries this is strictly prohibited.
Who makes the final decision on which drug is prescribed to a patient?	The prescribing physician is the only qualified to make such a decision with the diagnostic evidence in the patient file. Nevertheless you can ask the doctor about a new drug that you may have become aware of.
What is the patients' role in the decision?	As an empowered patient, you should be part of the decision, while taking into account the information your doctor provided, the information your pharmacists gave you, as well as the truthful information gathered elsewhere.
What if the drug I am prescribed does not work for me?	It may happen that your condition is not properly controlled by the medication you are prescribed and you may experience side effects that are very bothersome. In that case, you should go back to your doctor and see if there is a better option for you.

Chapter 9	Should you influence your doctor's decision on which drug to prescribe you?- Take away points (continuation)
Should I prepare for my next visit?	You may do some research yourself, and get familiar with the medications that can help you. There may even be a new drug in the market that you are willing to try since you do not feel better with what you are presently taking. Make a list of questions you want to ask your doctor during the next visit. I advise you to ask as many questions as you can. You should write the answers down if you need to remember important things.
What should the patient not do when interacting with a health professional	Do not challenge the doctors' knowledge. Do not be a ``wiki-patient`` .If you disagree, go elsewhere for a second opinion.
Should I request the doctor a specific drug?	You should not request for a specific drug, especially if your doctor does not believe that it is the best and safest option. Your doctor is liable for your prescription, and he/she will write it to the best of their ability.

Chapter 9	Should you influence your doctor's decision on which drug to prescribe you?- Take away points (continuation)
In which unique scenarios should a patient be firm in asking for a specific prescription?	If you are comfortable with your medication, it controls your symptoms well and you do not have bothersome side effects, but your doctor wants to change your prescription to a new one. You should ask to continue with the drug that is already working for you, unless specific reasons. If you were on the brand name of the product (called the originator drug) and your doctor is changing you to the generic alternative because it is cheaper or because the insurance will only pay for the cheapest generic alternative. In that case, if you feel uncomfortable with the change, be firm and pay for the difference.
What happens if the drug you are on is either discontinued, or in shortage?	The choices are to try a generic alternative or a similar originator drug from another company.

10

Your prescription and your *quality of life*

The effectiveness and safety of a prescription drug are assessed in clinical trials in order to support a market application, and in order for the drug to get approved by the regulators. In most of the cases, the data collected in those trials have to do with how the drug improved a particular symptom like high blood pressure or cholesterol levels in plasma, something that is measured objectively. A doctor who was selected as the principal investigator in a clinical trial measured the blood pressure of the patients on whom the drug was tested. During the clinical trial he/she was mostly focused on making sure that the objectives of the study are met, as for instance blood pressure control. Little time was dedicated to figure out how that control of blood pressure, or cholesterol for example, did improve the patient's quality of life. Mainly, patient input was not required because it was not a requirement for market approval. The approach of limited and focused observations is a thing from the past now. Evidence gathered through the years demonstrated that new drugs have to bring something better than only to control symptoms with some discomfort (side effects) to be successful in the market. Those new drugs have to really be better from what we have now. And who is better that the patients themselves to tell us their side of the story. Basically, we needed to know if the patients had their blood pressure controlled, but what it meant to them in terms of being able to perform their daily activities. How did they feel once the pressure was brought under control, is that a sustained control, or are there are ups and downs, is the drug helping to reduce the stress and anxiety of high blood pressure allowing the patient focus better in life, etc. Did the drug allowed the patient to resume his or her normal daily activities....and so on and so forth.....That new reporting approach is called PRO (*Patient Reported Outcomes*) where the patient plays a key role in clinical trial data reporting.

It is the patient who now becomes the focus of the research and not the new drug. This concept of health care is called "*patient centered or focused care*", meaning that you are the focus of the care and the treatment, and thus it is going to be tailored to your needs, in accordance with your requirements and characteristics (personalized medicine).

Presently, the focus is on *quality of life*, not only efficacy and safety. I will spend some time elaborating the concept in order to make you, the patient, aware of what we mean by that, and of what questions you will be asked by your doctor or pharmacist, or better, which answers they are seeking to obtain from you.

When we assess the *quality of life* of a patient, we take into account many things such as their physical, mental, psychological, economic and spiritual well-being. We do that utilizing validated questionnaires (validated means that they were tested and work as intended). Those questionnaires allow us to ask the same questions to everyone and provide all patients with the same set of possible answers. For example, one question can be as follows:

Q. On a scale from 1 (no pain) to 10 (the worst pain) please tell us how was your back pain in the last week in function of your daily life?

a) 0-2, no or minimal pain did not interfere with daily life

b) 3-5 some pain, minimally interfere with daily life

c) 6-8 moderate pain, interfered with daily life

d) 9-10 severe pain, daily life was completely disturbed

The response to this question will depend on many things as, for example, how the person perceives their pain, if he/she is taking any pain-killers or relaxants or other drugs that may interfere with the perception.

Basically, people can have different opinions on their quality of life, depending on what they are used to do, their socio-economic status, if they are employed or not, etc.

Good quality of life is something we all are aiming at. We want to live better, have longer and healthier lives, be independent, and a useful member of the society. The pharmaceutical industry, together with great advances in medicine, has improved our quality of life immensely. We live longer and better lives than our grandparents. But increase in length, i.e. longevity, is not necessarily a reflection of an increase in the quality of life. Quality of life may mean different things to all of us. I may feel better if I can drive, read, write, think and converse as well as if I can be physically fit and strong, earn a living, live, love.....

However, quality of life may mean something different to other people. Like for instance, someone may love to knit. However the rheumatoid arthritis does not allow them to do it, and therefore all other things may matter less.

To summarize, it is important that all your prescriptions have the ability not only to control your symptoms, but also to increase your quality of life, having minimal side effects or none at all, so you can normalize your own quality of life, whatever it means to you. Efficacy of a drug should be for you for instance, that your blood pressure is normal all day. Safety for you should be that, if there are any side effects, they do not disturb your daily life nor compromise your health and wellbeing. In that way, the medication should take you back to the most normal health status possible.

Chapter 10	Your prescription and your quality of life - Take away points
Why the focus has changed in the profile of new drugs?	Evidence gathered through the years demonstrated that new drugs have to bring something better than only to control symptoms with some discomfort (side effects) to be successful in the market.
What is quality of life assessment?	When we assess the quality of life of a patient, we take into account many things such as their physical, mental, psychological, economic and spiritual well-being. We do that utilizing validated questionnaires. People can have different opinions on their quality of life, depending on what they are used to do, their socio-economic status, if they are employed or not, etc.
The new reporting approach of clinical trials data is called PRO (Patient Reported Outcomes) where the patient plays a key role in clinical trial data reporting.	To assess the characteristics of a new drug, we needed to know if the patients had e.g. their blood pressure controlled, but also what it meant to them in terms of being able to perform their daily activities. How did they feel once the pressure was brought under control, is that a sustained control, or are there ups and downs, etc. Did the drug allowed the patient to resume his or her normal daily activities....and so on and so forth....

Chapter 10	Your prescription and your quality of life - Take away points (continuation)
What is patient centered or focused research/care?	It is the patient who now becomes the focus of the research and not the new drug. Meaning that you are the focus of the care and the treatment, and thus it is going to be tailored to your needs, in accordance with your requirements and characteristics (personalized medicine).
The new focus on prescription medication	Your prescriptions should have the ability not only to control your symptoms, but also to increase your quality of life, having minimal side effects or none at all, so you can normalize your own quality of life, whatever it means to you.

11

The importance of the right dose and dosage regimen

Previously, I mentioned how the axiom of the pharmaceutical industry used to be: 'one size fits all", and how far from the truth that was. When we talk about a *dose*, we refer to the amount of drug that has to be taken each time you use your medication. Generally, medications come in solid oral forms, i.e. pills that you can take by mouth without any intervention from a health professional.

Actually, the solid oral form is the preferred *dosage form*, since it is simple, portable, and easy to take, and as such is mostly accepted by patients and health professionals.

When a doctor prescribes a medication, he or she will specify to you which amount to take. The specified amount of your drug will most often be the one that is generally recommended in product specifications (SmPC Summary of Product Characteristics, or the Product Monograph that contains all the necessary information for the health professional) as the either *starting dose* or *optimal dose*.

Normally, the drug manufacturer will determine through RTC (randomized controlled clinical trials) the dose range in function of the desired response, which, too, will be within safety parameters. Within that range, they will select the minimum possible dose the patient has to take in order to have the best possible response with the minimum of adverse events. This way, you will achieve a reasonable therapeutic effect. That dose is established generally as the same for all adult subjects. Dose adjustments are seldom recommended unless concerns regarding safety and efficacy have been determined in clinical trials.

The other factor of safety in medication use is *dosage*. The drug manufacturer determines from the data in clinical trials how many times per day the drug has to be taken so as to maintain the desired effect safely. That will depend on the properties of the drug, and on human physiology.

Moreover, the *length of treatment* needs to be established, and that is done having in mind the disease itself, and the safety and efficacy of the product. Some drugs developed to control conditions like hypertension, are expected to be taken for life since they cannot cure the underlying condition. In cases like that, a limited time of treatment duration cannot be determined, and the prescription will be repeated.

For other conditions, like an ear infection, you will have a prescription written for treatment duration of a few days, but never exceeding a limited period of time, until the infection is cured.

There are certain drugs that you will use by taking a dose on an "as needed basis" (like puffers for asthma or painkillers for a headache).

Therefore, *dose, dosage regimen and length of treatment* are all important variables of drug safety, and as such are determined by the manufacturer. The doses that will be recommended are those considered reasonably safe and efficacious. If you reduce the recommended dose, regimen or length of treatment, you risk having an inefficacious treatment, adverse events, or a worsening of your condition that also represents a big risk. On the other hand, if you increase your recommended dose, regimen or length of treatment, you risk a toxic effect that could be very serious.

Since the dose, dosage regimen and length of treatment have been experimentally determined for each drug, the recommended amount is set in order to keep the patient safe and allow a reasonable therapeutic effect. Since the value is calculated based on the best response from the safety perspective, as observed in clinical trials on an ideal patient population, as we have already discussed, the recommended dose may not conform to your individual medical needs. This is where there is room for you to develop adverse events or be a *non-responder*. That will depend on the individual physiology and pharmacological factors. This is the reason why you should have your doctor adjust doses or modify prescriptions until you find the drug and the dose that suits your particular therapeutic needs.

Although I may have made my case against the 'one size fits all' approach, let us not forget that there is another reality, and that is that you must follow your doctor's instructions regarding the prescribed medication and that should keep you away from harm. You should not alter the dose or dosage regimen without consulting your doctor, because you may either overdose or under-dose, which can be very dangerous to your health.

Chapter 11	The importance of the right dose and dosage regimen from the safety perspective - Take away points
What do we mean by dose?	Dose is the amount of drug that has to be taken each time you use your medication. The doses that will be recommended are those considered reasonably safe and efficacious.
What is a dosage form?	Dosage form is the format that the manufacturer decided to make the drug in. Solid oral as a tablet, inject-able, topical cream, etc.
What is the dosage regimen?	The drug manufacturer determines from the data in clinical trials how many times per day the drug has to be taken so as to maintain the de-sired effect safely. That will depend on the properties of the drug, and on human physiology.
What is length of treatment?	The length of treatment (for how long you should take the therapy) needs to be established, and that is done having in mind the disease itself, and the safety and efficacy of the product.

12

Compliance to treatment, a challenge to achieve optimal therapeutic effect

Compliance is the measure of how well you conformed to the instructions provided to you regarding the proper use of your prescription medication.

Some of the biggest problems related to drug therapies do not always lie in the drugs themselves, but are caused by patients not following properly the instructions provided.

Poor compliance means that the patient did not take all the doses or follow the length of treatment needed to achieve the expected therapeutic effect. The reasons for poor compliance can be various.

One reason why a patient is not compliant, has to do more with 'health culture' as I call it, by which I consider that there is often a limited understanding among patients on the need to take their medication exactly as prescribed to treat their condition. This is all the more true in cases of illnesses that, if left untreated, in the long run, can become life threatening.

Another reason can be purely economic. The patient reduces the amount of medication, not understanding the risk of under-dosing. This usually results in a reduced efficacy of the drug, and an increase in the length of treatment, or in the need for more doctor follow-ups and sometimes even prescription changes.

The third reason for lack of compliance may be that the manufacturer established too many daily doses, some of which fall during the sleep time, making it impossible for the patient to strictly follow the regime. Then, they simply give up.

As you see, the more doses you have to take in a day, the less compliant you will be, thus putting your therapeutic benefit at risk.

The fourth compliance issue, related to the one previously described, is that patients tend to squeeze a dosage regimen of 3 or more times a day during wake hours, thus increasing the amount of drug circulating in blood to levels that could become dangerous.

For instance, if you have to take 3 doses of amoxicillin, of 500 mg each, you are supposed to take one every 8 hours. However, if you squeeze those 1.5 grams of daily total over some 16 wake hours, it means that you will have an increase of at least 50% in the amount of amoxicillin circulating in your bloodstream during the day, and that could result in a serious safety issue and trigger toxicity.

Thanks to the fact that amoxicillin is safe even when the dose is increased by 50%, this particular example may not represent a real risk in case of failure to comply.

However, if I were to choose theophylline, or carbamazepine, drugs that have what is called a *narrow therapeutic index* (meaning that the dose window where the drug is therapeutic is very small, not allowing dose changes without compromising safety), you are potentially risking serious side effects.

The fifth reason behind the lack of compliance is no efficacy. The drug may not work for you (you are a non-responder), and therefore you start skipping doses, or giving up. However, this is a case where we must evaluate the situation very carefully. Certain drugs exert their intended therapeutic effect immediately after being taken, as are pain relievers or diuretics. When the drug is discontinued, the therapeutic effect disappears as well. Conversely, there are certain drugs that are not so straightforward. Take for instance antidepressants (especially the ones called SSRIs-selective serotonin reuptake inhibitors) in the case of which you have to take the medication for several weeks until you are able to observe some therapeutic effect. That is due to the fact that the therapeutic effect is mediated though intracellular processes involving protein synthesis. That kind of drugs where you have to wait for a long time for a therapeutic effect, are and ideal candidate for noncompliance since the expected benefit may not be perceived in a short period of time and the patient might give up.

Therefore, patients should be warned of what to expect when a new drug is introduced, and written information, provided by the pharmacist, should be readily available for patient's review.

Remember that you should always consult your health care provider or pharmacist before making any change in your medication.

Chapter 12	Compliance to treatment, a challenge to achieve optimal therapeutic effect - Take away points
What is compliance to treatment?	Compliance is the measure of how well you conformed to the instructions provided to you regarding the proper use of your prescription medication.
Reasons for lack of compliance	-'Health culture' as I call it, by which I consider is that there is often a limited understanding among patients on the need to take their medication exactly as prescribed to treat their condition. -Second, can be purely financial. - Third, for lack of compliance may be that the manufacturer established too many daily doses, some of which fall during the sleep time, making it impossible for the patient to strictly follow the regime. - Fourth, related to the one previously described, is that patients tend to squeeze a dosage regimen of 3 or more times a day during wake hours, thus increasing the amount of drug circulating in blood to levels that could become dangerous -The fifth reason behind the lack of compliance is efficacy. The drug may not work for you (you are a non-responder), and therefore you start skipping doses, or giving up.

Chapter 12	Compliance to treatment, a challenge to achieve optimal therapeutic effect - Take away points (continuation)
How to promote drug compliance?	Patients should be warned of what to expect when a new drug is introduced, and written information, provided by the pharmacist, should be readily available for patient's review

13

Dosing and taking drugs of special pharmacology

Certain drugs cannot be introduced at the optimal therapeutic dose at once. One of the reasons for it is because your body has to learn how to deal with the drug, and slowly adapt to its presence in order to respond as expected. Your doctor will introduce certain drugs slowly, increasing the dose weekly, or at longer intervals, until achieving the optimal dose. That process is called *titration*. It is very important that you follow the process because you may experience serious side effects otherwise. Drugs that must be titrated also have to be discontinued slowly, since any abrupt discontinuation may precipitate serious adverse symptoms and you may end up in the emergency room. That kind of discontinuation process is called *weaning off*. In the case that you have to change this type of medications in the middle of the treatment, you must follow the special regimen for switching therapies, as indicated by your doctor, to avoid the occurrence of any serious adverse event. The type of drugs that may need titration and weaning off are generally CNS drugs (those acting at the level of the central nervous system, as antidepressants, seizure medications, anxiolytics, antipsychotic medication, and the like). Always ask your doctor about the drug dosage if you are taking any of these medications. Never discontinue on your own, and always listen to your body. If anything seems to be unusual, consult your health care provider immediately.

Chapter 13	Dosing and taking drugs of special pharmacology- Take away points
What is titration?	Your doctor will introduce certain drugs slowly, increasing the dose weekly, or at longer intervals, until achieving the optimal dose. That process is called titration.
What is weaning off?	Drugs that must be titrated also have to be discontinued slowly, since any abrupt discontinuation may precipitate serious adverse symptoms and you may end up in the emergency room
How do you change special pharmacology drug therapies?	In the case that you have to change this type of medications in the middle of the treatment, you must follow the special regimen for switching therapies, as indicated by your doctor, to avoid the occurrence of any serious adverse event. The process is tailored according to the drugs involved.

14

Other important safety concerns you should be aware of

You must be aware that the use of any medication comes with a risk, as we have previously discussed. Some medication can be more risky than others because of its toxic profile. You should be very vigilant with side effects and always consult with your doctor or pharmacist when you notice an unusual symptom developing, regardless of how long you have been taking the medication.

There are several safety issues that you should pay attention to. This applies especially if you are taking certain medications with *boxed warnings* (this is a type of warning introduced by the FDA to warn about serious safety concerns identified linked to the use of a particular drug), or with known safety concerns that require caution.

The first important safety issue I am going to discuss is *overdose*. At therapeutic doses, overdosing is extremely rare, unless it becomes a result of a drug interaction, which I am going to discuss later. Overdose means that the patient took a larger than the safe maximum tolerated dose determined in clinical trials, and therefore developed serious adverse drug reactions that may result in a life threatening situation.

Overdose may result from unintentional consumption of larger amounts of a drug, as a result of misunderstanding the right dosing, or just because you forgot you had already taken your drug and took it again.

Earlier in the book I mentioned Paracelsus and his rationale that anything can be toxic, and that the only thing that differentiates a remedy from a poison is the dose.

You can even overdose on water if you drink huge amounts of it, momentarily diluting your blood and body fluids decompensating[9] all your body functions.

Another type of overdose is intentional, when large amounts of drugs are taken on purpose.

The second safety concern is *dependency*. Dependency occurs when you need to take more medication irrespective of the therapeutic need. In general, drugs that may create the risk of dependency are properly labelled and warnings are written to make both the doctor and the patient aware of this possibility. Well-determined protocols for dosing, use, and weaning or discontinuation are developed and provided to minimize this risk. The majority of opioid[10]-related painkillers can pose this risk. Also other drugs that act at the level of the central nervous system might create dependency. The risk is higher if you have alcohol or other chemical dependencies. You must always consult with your doctor about the issue. Inquire about a non-addictive alternative, if available, to treat your condition, if you consider that dependency may be a real problem.

---

[9] Decompensation may occur when the blood composition including electrolytes, proteins as well as blood cells is pathologically altered.

[10] Opioids are a family of drugs related to opium as are oxycontin, oxycodone, oxyneo, morphine among others

In my opinion, opioid-based painkillers like Percocet™, are too often prescribed for minor conditions like pains and strains caused by sports activities, minor injuries or simple surgery.

Again, you as a patient are ultimately responsible for your health and well-being, and therefore should make an informed decision before taking any medication that is known to produce dependency.

Another very important safety issue is *lack of efficacy,* where the drug is not working as it is expected. Drugs that are marketed are those that have demonstrated an acceptable rate of efficacy in treating a particular condition in the general population. That efficacy was demonstrated in controlled clinical trials. However, demonstrating efficacy in clinical trials is one thing, and being efficient in the market is another. This brings us now to another concept and that is *efficiency*.

A drug is considered efficient when the physician prescribing it is able to replicate the effect demonstrated in clinical trials on his patients in the clinic. The level of efficiency varies depending on one, the diagnostic precision of the prescribing physician and two, the dose provided to the patient. What I mean is that if you do not have the disease the drug intends to treat, you may not feel any benefit, but share all the risks. Also, if the dose is incorrect, the drug may not provide you all the therapeutic benefit it is intended to.

Basically, to avoid the *lack of efficacy*, the prescribing physician should prescribe the right drug, and for the right condition, as described in the labelling of the product, and at the right dose. That dose will be initially recommended by the manufacturer of the drug. In addition, to make the most appropriate prescription, the physician must take into account your allergies, other underlying diseases (kidney or liver impairments), and any other medications and supplements you may be taking.

Unfortunately, the economic factor also plays a key role in prescribing drugs. The type of medication your doctor will prescribe you tends to be tailored to various factors. For example, instead of the drug you may benefit the best, your doctor may prescribe you another similar drug that is covered by insurers, or a drug with the cheapest generic alternatives, which may not necessarily be the most efficacious therapy for your condition, and may keep you sick for longer or just not at best that you could be.

Also, the possibility exists that the generic alternative you are dispensed at a given time is not as good as the previous one, in which case you will feel the difference in efficacy. Always consult your doctor if you feel that the drug you are taking may not be working for you, which, as we have discussed previously in the book, may be due to many factors.

Allergies are a serious safety concern when any medical intervention is proposed. If you are aware of your own allergies to certain drugs or foods, those have to be very well established and communicated to your doctor. However, you may have allergies to certain things that you are not aware of, or develop a new allergy to a drug you may be presently taking. You should always be vigilant, especially when you have a history of allergy, and report any unusual rash, skin reaction, and swelling of eyelids or lips. Quickly go to your doctor or go to the nearest ER if you develop shortness of breath, swelling or other serious allergic symptoms. Allergies can be fatal since they can evolve into a serious situation in minutes.

There is also the possibility of *drug, food or nutritional supplement interactions* that can become a serious safety issue. Anything you take has the potential to interact with the medication you are prescribed. The reason is very simple. Our livers are responsible for cleaning our body from toxic and foreign substances in order to keep the balance in the body. That cleaning is done through chemical reactions catalyzed by our own enzymes. Drugs, supplements as well as certain food components may share the same enzymatic pathway for metabolism and may be responsible for inhibiting or inducing enzymes in charge of metabolising other drugs making the metabolic process different.

And that is the tale of drug interactions.

Let's assume you are taking two drugs at the same time because you need them to control two different conditions or problems you have. The first interaction scenario can be that, whilst your liver is occupied cleaning the body form one drug, those enzymes are busy, and therefore cannot clean the body from the second drug or from the supplement you may be taking, because they happen to share the same enzyme for metabolism. In turn, the second drug you took starts to accumulate in your body dangerously towards toxic levels and you could end up with a serious drug reaction. Another scenario may happen when, due to interactions between drugs, one drug inhibits an enzyme responsible for activating the metabolism of the other drug you are taking, and therefore the other drug becomes inefficacious. If that other drug was for example a drug to control your blood pressure, you may be exposed to a serious risk due to lack of efficacy caused by the said drug interaction. Minerals like calcium, magnesium and others, as well as herbal medicines and vitamins may play a big role in drug interactions. Always consult your doctor or pharmacists about this issue and make sure that you took note of all supplements you are taking, including the morning grapefruit.

A very common interaction concern is the one between oral contraceptives and other medication the patient may need to treat a condition, which may make an oral contraceptive inefficient and therefore produce an unplanned pregnancy.

This brings me to the topic of *pregnancy* and pharmacotherapy. Pregnant women should avoid the use of any medication to reduce the risk of harming the embryo/fetus. The thalidomide disaster of the sixties is the book case for any doubt about the issue where pregnant women were prescribed the drug to control morning sickness yielding children with serious limb malformations due to catastrophic fetal effects. Moreover, pregnant women should refrain from alcohol, cigarettes and the so called recreational drugs. Clinical trials are NOT conducted in pregnant women, and they are explicitly excluded from clinical research due to ethical and moral reasons. Consequently, we lack enough information on the safety of drugs in human pregnancy.

Nevertheless, there may be a case when pregnant women are the indicated population for a particular drug in a clinical trial, in which case they are allowed entry. Also, some drugs may have human pregnancy data since women may unknowingly become pregnant during the clinical study and were then followed up to determine the effect of the accidental exposure to the tested drug on the embryo/ foetus.

Pregnant women or women who want to become pregnant may have serious underlying health conditions which necessitate continuous treatment, such as epilepsy. In those cases, the patient should talk to the doctor before thinking about becoming pregnant, since the pregnancy safety of antiepileptic drugs is well established, and the women may need to be switched to safer options to avoid harming the unborn child. Sometimes a safer alternative is not possible, and you should be very aware of it. Also, other medications that you may consider safe as are over-the-counter medications for flu, cough syrups, anti-allergy drugs, anti-nausea medication and many others, may not be safe to use during pregnancy. Herbal remedies and supplements fall also under this category. Always consult with your doctor if you are pregnant or

125

planning to become pregnant about the safety of the drugs you have to take. Also, breastfeeding should be avoided during drug therapy, because the majority of the marketed drugs may be present in breast-milk owing it to their ability to pass through tissues and membranes.

A distinctive safety concern I am going to write about is the one involving drugs and *special populations*. The 'special populations' are people who are either too young (children) or too old (elderly) or have serious conditions or diseases that make them metabolize or eliminate drugs differently than what has been established in the sample population tested in clinical trials. Not all the liver enzymes are completely active in newborns and infants. In children and elderly people, the liver enzymes work at different velocities than in the general population, and have different affinities for their substrates. People referred to as liver- (hepatic) or kidney- (renal) impaired have altered the mechanisms that control the level of drugs in blood due to their condition. They are prone to two serious types of adverse drug reactions as are overdosing (toxicity) due to limited clearance[11] from the body, or lack of efficacy due to inability

[11] Drug clearance is a pharmacokinetic measure of the body's ability to clear the drug from blood by all body systems

to metabolize the drug to an active form, or the body just clears the drug untouched. These impairments affect the bioavailability[12] of the drug to make the treatment efficacious.

In all these cases, if suggested by the drug manufacturer, dose adjustments should be made to avoid a seriously detrimental reaction.

If the drug manufacturer hasn't explicitly recommended dose adjustments for such cases, it is the doctor who should reconsider dose adjustments.

Lastly, but not less important, I am going to talk about *suicidality*. There has been a lot of discussion about suicidality and antidepressants. Drugs can affect the brain and how we think to such an extent that suicidality and also homicidality[13] can be developed. The FDA has requested just recently, for suicidality to be determined in clinical trials as a potential safety concern, regardless of the indication for the drug studied. Although suicidali-

---

[12] Drug bioavailability refer to the amount of drug available in the body to produce effects at the target site

[13] Homicidality could become a drug related adverse event where due to the central nervous acting nature of the drug, the patient develops a paranoid ideation and/or compulsion to hurt another human being.

ty is potentially a serious safety concern, it must be very well established before a boxed warning is issued. You should be very vigilant with drugs with this kind of warnings, and if you have to take medications with this established potential effect, you ought to follow doctor's instructions and a good idea is not to live alone during the treatment period.

Chapter 14	Other important safety concerns you should be aware of - Take away points
What is a boxed warning?	This is a type of warning introduced by the FDA to warn about serious safety concerns identified linked to the use of a particular drug.
What is overdose?	Overdose means that the patient took a larger than the safe maximum tolerated dose determined in clinical trials, and therefore developed serious adverse drug reactions that may result in a life threatening situation.
How can you overdose?	Overdose may result from unintentional consumption of larger amounts of a drug, as a result of misunderstanding the right dosing, or just because you forgot you had already taken your drug and took it again.
What is dependency?	Dependency occurs when you need to take more medication irrespective of the therapeutic need.
What does lack of efficacy mean for you?	That the prescribed drug does not work as intended and therefore your condition is not controlled.
What is efficiency?	A drug is considered efficient when the physician prescribing it is able to replicate the effect demonstrated in clinical trials on his patients in the clinic. The level of efficiency varies depending on the diagnostic precision of the prescribing physician and two, the dose provided to the patient.

Chapter 14	Other important safety concerns you should be aware of - Take away points (continuation)
What happens if you have allergies?	Allergies are a serious safety concern when any medical intervention is proposed. If you are aware of your own allergies to certain drugs or foods, those have to be very well established and communicated to your doctor.
Can drug interactions become a problem for your new prescription?	There is also the possibility of drug, food or nutritional supplement interactions that can become a serious safety issue. Anything you take has the potential to interact with the medication you are prescribed. Drugs, supplements as well as food components may share the same enzymatic pathway for metabolism and may be responsible for inhibiting or inducing enzymes in charge of metabolising other drugs making the metabolic process different.
What if you become pregnant during drug therapy?	Pregnant women should avoid the use of any medication to reduce the risk of harming the embryo/fetus. Moreover, pregnant women should refrain from alcohol, cigarettes and the so called recreational drugs. Clinical trials are NOT conducted in pregnant women, and they are explicitly excluded from clinical research due to ethical and moral reasons.

Chapter 14	Other important safety concerns you should be aware of - Take away points (continuation)
What are special populations?	The 'special populations' are people who are either too young (children) or too old (elderly) or have serious conditions or diseases that make them metabolize or eliminate drugs differently than what has been established in the sample population tested in clinical trials.
What is suicidality?	It is the adverse event described as suicide intent or completion due to the effect of a therapeutic product. Suicidality has been initially reported with the use of antidepressants, especially in the vulnerable group of adolescents, and become a boxed warning for these medications.
What does homicidality mean?	Homicidality could become a drug related adverse event where due to the central nervous acting nature of the drug, the patient develops a paranoid ideation and/or compulsion to hurt another human being.

131

15

What you should know about dosage forms

The medications you may be prescribed may come in many different dosage forms[14].

As I have already mentioned, the industry aims at developing solid oral forms (the 'magic pills') to allow patients to self-administer their medication without a need for an intervention by a professional.

Solid oral forms are easy to use, easily portable, readily available, and simple.

They can come as pills, tablets, capsules, soft gels, you name it. The drug dosage is limited and easy to control.

---

[14]It's the form the manufacturer decides to make the drug (tablet, syrup, injectable, etc.)

Another oral intake form you are probably very familiar with is the liquid form, as are syrups, extracts, oils and the likes. In general, these forms are provided in bottles. Most children drugs are produced in liquids since kids do not fare well taking pills or capsules. A liquid form allows you more control over the dosage, since you can vary the volume and hence the dose necessary. Their big advantage, however, is that, since they do not require being dissolved in the gut, their action is faster. For example, when it comes to pain relievers, I personally prefer liquid forms, because their action is very fast. On the other hand, liquid forms have a shorter shelf life, and are very impractical for transportation.

In one word, oral forms are any drugs that are delivered by mouth. Note that puffers do not belong to this group because they are intended to access the lungs and therefore belong to another delivery form group.

The scientific name for oral forms is *enteral* (Greek 'enteron' means intestine, or digestive system).

Another delivery form that is enteral, but not very common are suppositories, these are delivered through the anal cavity, and therefore not favoured unless necessary. They are however very useful in infants or people that cannot take medication by mouth.

There is another form that is called *parenteral* (Greek 'para', besides and 'enteros' intestines, referring to the drugs that are not delivered through the digestive tract, 'enteron'). Parenteral are drugs that are delivered intravenously, intra-arterially, subcutaneously or intramuscularly. Most of the injections administered to patients using needles are parenterals. Most of the parenteral drugs are administered by needles. You may be familiar with them since vaccines are generally delivered by subcutaneous or intramuscular injections.

Other medications that cannot be taken by mouth due to many reasons are delivered in this way. In general, we need a health care provider to administer the parenterals, and therefore there is an added cost for delivery. However, there are exceptions to this rule. The best known exceptions are insulin and the EpiPen™, which patients usually administer themselves.

Both parenteral and enteral forms aim to reach the blood stream and then to reach the site of action from there. That is why they are called drugs of *systemic action*. Puffers, patches, and certain creams, even though they seem to be local or topical, are, in fact, systemic by nature. That means that they enter through lungs or skin, but they reach the entire body.

Just as there are systemic drugs, that will access the entire body through the blood stream, there are also *topical drugs*, which are intended to act locally where applied. Those are local antibiotic, antifungal and anti-allergic creams and gels as well as local pain relievers. They are very commonly used and generally available over the counter. You have to be aware that the topicals, besides acting locally, also get absorbed into the body and can be found in very small amounts in the bloodstream. Therefore, patients must be very careful and follow doctor's and manufacturer's instructions.

There also exists a myriad of novel delivery forms to improve the therapeutic potential/performance of a drug. All of them are aimed to deliver the right amount of highly active medication, and, at the same time, to reduce the adverse events to the least possible measure. See table 3-Drug Delivery Forms Simplified.

Table 3 – Drug delivery forms simplified			
Action	**Delivery route**	**Type**	**Examples**
Systemic (the entire body)	Enteral	oral	Tablets, capsules, pills, solutions, syrups, extracts, etc.
		anal	Suppositories, creams, gels, etc.
Systemic (the entire body)	Parenteral	i.v.	Intra-venous injection
		i.m.	Intra-muscular injection
		i.a.	Intra-arterial injection
		topical	Patches, gels, creams, oils, etc.
		pulmonary	Puffers, inhalation sprays, etc.
Local (localized area)	Local	Topical	Gels, creams, powders, foams, sprays, etc.

Chapter 15	What you should know about dosage forms Take away points
Dosage form	It's the form the manufacturer decides to make the drug (tablet, syrup, injectable, etc.)
Which is the preferred dosage form and why?	The pharmaceutical industry aims at developing solid oral forms (the 'magic pills') to allow patients to self-administer their medication without a need for an intervention by a professional.
What are the advantages of solid oral forms?	Solid oral forms are easy to use, easily portable, readily available, and simple. They can come as pills, tablets, capsules, soft gels, you name it. The drug dosage is limited and easy to control.
What is the most common dosage form for children medications?	Most children drugs are produced in liquids since kids do not fare well taking pills or capsules. A liquid form allows you more control over the dosage, since you can vary the volume and hence the dose necessary.
Are all topically applied drugs are intended to work locally?	A topical form is not always developed to act locally. Topical forms can be developed to deliver systemic drugs as are nicotine or hormone based patches.
Are all drugs delivered pulmonary intended to treat the lungs?	No, the respiratory system has become the target to easily deliver drugs that have the intention to act systemically, as are insulin inhalers.

16

Off-label use of marketed drugs

In the last 25 years, the field of pharmaco-therapeutics has made great advances rendering diseases once untreatable, as HIV-Aids and Hepatitis C, treatable as chronic conditions.

Drugs and nutritional supplements have enhanced our health and well-being and have greatly improved our quality of life.

Generally, to address a disease or condition, doctors prescribe drugs or therapeutic interventions considered of benefit to patients. In most cases, drugs are prescribed according to approved indications, and their safety and efficacy has been well established in controlled clinical trials.

But despite the fact that there is quite a number of drugs in the market to treat commonly known conditions as hypertension, high cholesterol or diabetes, many other conditions are poorly addressed by marketed drugs within their established indications[15]. So the public belief that 'there is a pill for every ill' is unfortunately erroneous. Doctors are left powerless when they encounter a patient with a condition as for example autism in their practice, and there is little relief available for them to offer to the patient, because neither the aetiology of the disease is understood, nor a therapy has been established to treat it.

As previously discussed in this book, drugs are able to trigger many responses or effects owing to their ability to bind to specific receptors on the cell surface. By doing so, they trigger further intracellular reactions that are ultimately observed as either therapeutic effects or side effects in the clinic trial. Those effects are presented as the pharmacological effects of a drug. The so called primary pharmacology of a drug is defined by the main therapeutic effect observed in the drug which at the same time has market importance. All other potential therapeutic effects that the drug may have presented but are not as important or are of a lesser market importance are considered secondary pharmacology of the drug.

---

[15] uses approved for marketing and sale

Lastly, there are "unwanted" effects that a drug may produce due to its pleiotropic nature (acts at the level of many cells and tissues producing widespread effects), that we define as "side effects" or "adverse drug reactions".

If we look pragmatically at all the identified effects of a drug, the one most favoured and the main reason the drug is going to be developed is the one which is pharmacologically safe and has the greatest market potential.

In order to maximize the return on their investment, pharmaceutical companies register a drug listing the indication with the best market potential, while leaving all other potential uses out of the scope of the indication. Drugs are hence registered in one or more indications that make market sense. Simply put, to invest in developing a drug in an off-label indication just may not be profitable.

Therefore, to complete the concept, any time practitioners prescribe a drug away from its approved indication, they are using it "off-label".

In order to protect the health and wellbeing of the population, regulators prohibit pharmaceutical companies to market drugs away from the approved indications. Nevertheless, marketed drugs can be studied away from their indicated and approved use in the phase III of clinical trials, so as to further enhance the knowledge of their safety and efficacy and to support the applicability of available drugs to unmet needs.

As I have already pointed out, it is completely legal for doctors to prescribe drugs out of the scope of the original intended use or "off-label" to patients, if, in their qualified opinion, they consider that the drug may be of therapeutic benefit to the patient.

The main risk of the "off-label" use is that safety, as defined earlier in the book, was not determined in controlled clinical trials for the off-label population (i.e. it was not defined by age group, gender, disease, dose and dosage regimens, underlying diseases, concomitant medications, etc.). Therefore, the risk can be considerable since there are many new unknowns in the drug profile for the off-label use.

Although the risks are evident, benefits can also be very tangible.

For instance, SSRIs (selective serotonin reuptake inhibitors) have several approved indications and are mainly known for the treatment of depression. However, there are at least six more "off-label" uses with different levels of evidence for safety and efficacy.

142

In conclusion, off-label use of drugs is part of standard practice in medicine that enables doctors to provide for treatments for unmet needs. There are potential risks when drugs are used off-label, as well as evident benefits. The prescribing physicians consider all possible options before deciding on prescribing a drug off-label. Patients benefit from the off-label use if their conditions are met.

Since today many people have access to Internet and can search for the approved uses of the drug they have been prescribed, patients may be surprised if they learn that their drug does not treat their symptoms. It is therefore important that patients be made aware of all the above described facts when they are prescribed a drug off-label.

Chapter 16	Off-label use of marketed drugs - Take away points
What is "off-label" use?	Any time practitioners prescribe a drug away from its approved indication, they are using it "off-label".
Are there risks for off-label use?	The main risk of the "off-label" use is that safety, as defined earlier in the book, was not determined in controlled clinical trials for the off-label population.
What are the benefits from off-label use?	Off-label use of drugs is part of standard practice in medicine that enables doctors to provide for treatments for unmet needs.
Why is it illegal for pharmaceutical companies to market a drug for off-label uses?	In order to protect the health and wellbeing of the population, regulators prohibit pharmaceutical companies to market drugs away from the approved indications.
Is it legal for doctors to prescribe drugs off-label?	It is completely legal for doctors to prescribe drugs out of the scope of the original intended use or "off-label" to patients, if, in their qualified opinion, they consider that the drug may be of therapeutic benefit to the patient.

17

Safety concerns about slow release/timed release/extended release forms

I would like to dedicate the last chapter of this book to bringing your awareness towards solid oral slow release forms. These dosage forms were created to reduce the number of doses of a drug a patient has to take in a day, and are designed to increase compliance and maintain the therapeutic effect in cases where small changes in blood concentration can have an adverse effect on the patients' wellbeing.

Slow /timed /extended release forms are created in such manner that a full day (or a longer period) amount of drug is available in one pill that a pa-

145

tient is to take daily or periodically as per their doctor's instructions. They are very convenient and increase compliance.

These solid forms are manufactured with the purpose of providing a single pill that must not be divided, or sliced, in any way. It is very important that you take the whole pill as it is provided by the manufacturer, since an entire days' worth of dose may be in there, if not more, and if the pill's integrity is damaged in any way, shape, or form, it may produce what is called *dose dumping*, and therefore you may end up having one entire day's worth of medication released inside your body all at once, instead of it being slowly delivered to you in the course of the day. That may produce serious toxic effects, even catastrophic/lethal ones, depending on the type of the drug the pill contained.

Never divide or tamper with a slow/ timed/ extended release form. If you are unsure of, or have any doubts regarding its integrity, do not take it but rather ask your pharmacist for further instructions.

These slow/extended/timed release forms are generally manufactured either with a mesh on the pill that dissolves slowly inside your digestive tract, making the drug slowly available during the day, or they are compressed into layers with different solubility patterns, or there might be some other type of release mechanism that will allow you to take the minimum number of pills in a day.

The safety of these delivery forms depends on the integrity and quality of the pill. Be very careful when handling them, and make sure that you follow your health care provider's instructions.

Enteric coated drugs are not the same as slow/ timed or extended released forms. They are drugs that were coated with special materials that do not dissolve in the stomach, reducing stomach upset, and serious gastrointestinal erosion. There drugs are intended to dissolve in the small intestine. Aspirin™ for example is marketed in enteric coated drug dosage forms. Also in this case you should not divide the tablet, since the coat is open and the drug is delivered in the stomach potentially producing serious adverse drug reactions.

Chapter 17	Safety concerns about slow release/timed release/extended release forms - Take away points
What are slow release/timed release/extended release forms?	They were created to reduce the number of doses of a drug a patient has to take in a day, and are designed to increase compliance and maintain the therapeutic effect in cases where small changes in blood concentration can have an adverse effect on the patients' wellbeing.
Are slow release / timed/extend release forms safe?	It the integrity of the tablet/pill is not affected, they have an acceptable safety profile.
Can you divide the slow release dose?	Never divide or tamper with a slow/timed/extended release form. It is very important that you take the whole pill as it is provided by the manufacturer, since an entire days' worth of dose may be in there, if not more, and if the pill's integrity is damaged in any way, shape, or form, it may produce what is called dose dumping, and therefore you may end up having one entire day's worth of medication released inside your body all at once, instead of it being slowly delivered to you in the course of the day.

Chapter 17	Safety concerns about slow release/timed release/extended release forms - Take away points (continuation)
What if I divide a slow release form?	It may produce serious toxic effects; even catastrophic/lethal ones depending on the type of the drug the pill contained dumping large amount of drugs at once.
Are slow release and enteric coating the same thing?	Enteric coated drugs are not the same as slow/ timed or extended released forms. They are drugs that were coated with special materials that do not dissolve in the stomach, reducing stomach upset, and serious gastrointestinal erosion.

18

Patient Centered Medicine vs. Patient Centric Medicine and vs. Personalized Medicine

In Clinical Research as in Medical Practice, there has been a flurry of misconceptions and misunderstanding of the concepts of Patient Centric Medicine, Patient Centered Medicine and Personalized Medicine. Some professionals use the terms interchangeably yielding to further puzzling in patients and others. Let me bring some light to the concepts, so everyone can be in the same page in the conversation.

Where all these new concepts do came from?

First, let's see why these concepts have been developed. Here I have some insights:

The main issue was how to implement new revolutionizing technologies to improve the way medical care is delivered efficiently.

Also, to give an insight to patients that they are going to be greatly benefited by new technologies and approaches to their care.

Lastly, to create a frame of work for scientists and governments in function of where the funds are going to go to achieve the first.

Basically, we needed to reinvent medicine and delivery of care to include those new technologies as key for great improvement.

Then, let's look at the concepts and how they affect medical care.

What is Patient Centered Medicine?

Going back in the history of the term, the Committee on Quality of Health Care in America, IOM, published a document titled " Crossing the Quality Chasm" A New Health Care system for the 21st. Century"(2001). This document coined the concept Patient-Centered Care as "providing care that is respectful of and responsive to individual patient preferences, needs, and values and ensuring that patient values guide all clinical decisions". Further, the NIH elaborated the term as "health care that establishes a partnership among practitioners, patients, and their families (when appropriate) to ensure that decisions respect patients' wants, needs and preferences and solicit patients' input on the education and support they need to make decisions and participate in their own care".

Basically, patient-centered medicine (care) involves the patient (and their families) in the decision of how care is delivered meanwhile key for that decision is to provide with accurate information and support.

What is Patient Centric Medicine?

Patient centric medicine is based on the fact that the patient is the source of the information and point of interaction for the delivery of care. This centricity is possible due to new technologies that allow patients to produce their own data easily and submit it directly to the health provider to guide the medical care decisions. In clinical research, that concept has been the key in data collection though electronic patient reported outcome systems (ePRO), to allow the ongoing collection of safety and efficacy data to proactively make near real time decisions on the subjects participation.

Patient centric medicine is based on the fact that the patient is the source of the information and point of interaction for the delivery of care.

It is important to know that the concept is unintentionally interchanged with patient centered medicine, especially when looking into the Affordable Care Act (US) and its interpretations.

What is Personalized Medicine?

Although the concept is not new, National Academy of Sciences (NAS) defines personalized medicine as "the use of genomic, epigenomic, exposure and other data to define individual patterns of disease, potentially leading to better individual treatment." It is used interchangeably as "precision medicine," "stratified medicine," "targeted medicine," and "pharmacogenomics," I personally like the concept of pharmacogenomics, whereas the analysis and identification of specific genomic markers would allow pinpoint the right medicine where the patient will respond and not have serious adverse events.

As you can see, they are three completely different concepts, that once well-defined and understood, it should allow its implementation to health care in a seamless manner.

Chapter 18	Patient Centered Medicine vs. Patient Centric Medicine and vs. Personalized Medicine –Take Away Points
Patient Centered Medicine (care)	Providing care that is respectful of and responsive to individual patient preferences, needs, and values and ensuring that patient values guide all clinical decisions
Patient Centric Medicine	Patient centric medicine is based on the fact that the patient is the source of the information and point of interaction for the delivery of care
Personalized Medicine	The use of genomic, epigenomic, exposure and other data to define individual patterns of disease, potentially leading to better individual treatment.

Notes

Notes

Notes

Notes